THE BEACH BODY DIET COOKBOOK

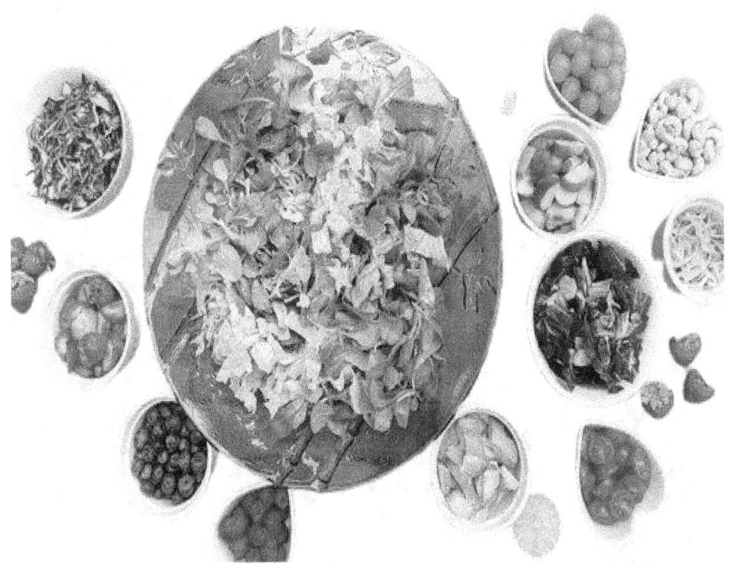

Dr. Mary Dixon

Copyright © 2023 by Dr. Penny Watson

All rights reserved. No part of this publication may be reproduced, distributed, or transmitted in any form or by any means, including photocopying, recording, or other electronic or mechanical methods, without the prior written permission of the publisher, except in the case of brief quotations embodied in critical reviews and certain other noncommercial uses permitted by copyright law.

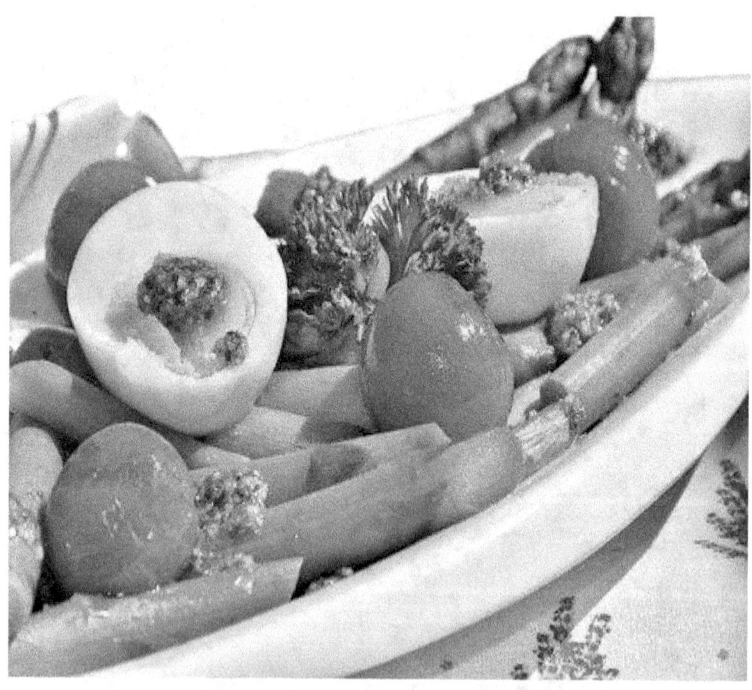

Table of Contents

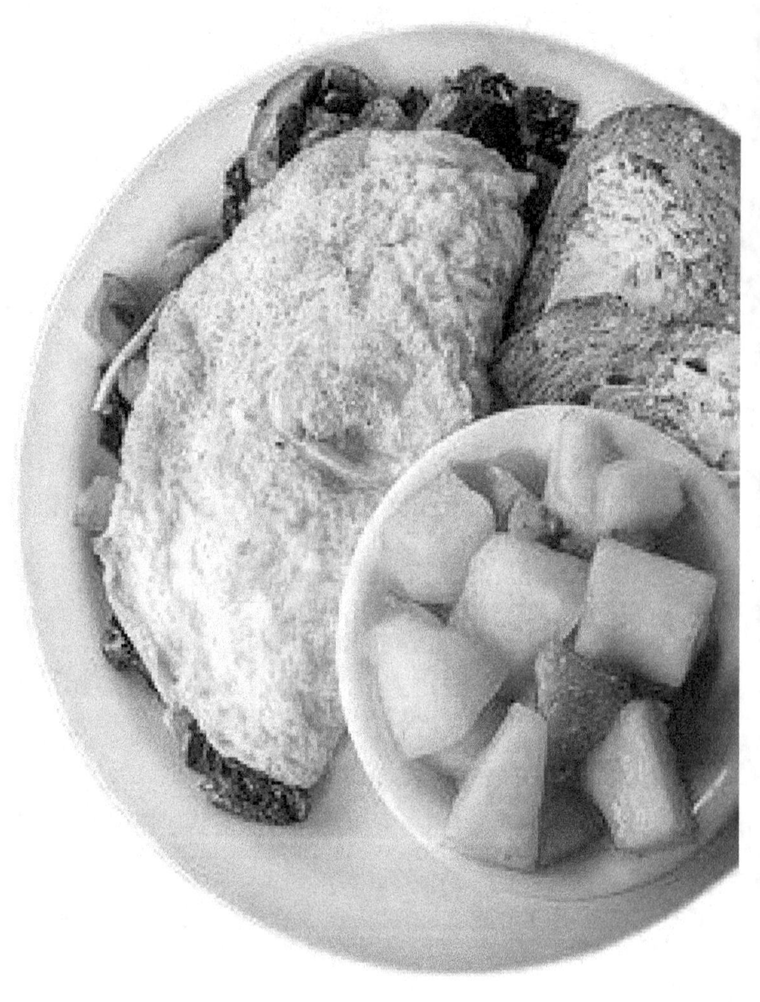

INTRODUCTION

Lena had always been self-conscious about her body, especially during the summer months when everyone seemed to be flaunting their beach-ready physiques. She had tried countless diets and exercise programs in the past, but nothing seemed to work.

One day, Lena stumbled upon a nutrition program that promised to help her achieve her dream body. She made the desperate decision to try it despite her doubts.

The first few days were tough as Lena had to cut out many of her favourite foods, but she stuck with it. As the days went by, she started noticing changes in her body. Her clothes were fitting better, and she had more energy.

A month into the program, Lena was amazed at the progress she had made. Her stomach was flatter, and her legs were leaner. She felt confident and proud of her body for the first time in years.

When summer arrived, Lena headed to the beach with her friends.

As she slipped into her swimsuit, she couldn't believe how good she looked. She strutted confidently along the beach, feeling like a whole new person.

At the end of the day, Lena collapsed onto her towel, exhausted but happy. She had achieved her beach body, and it was all thanks to the right diet. She realized that all those years of struggling with her body could have been avoided if she had only found the right program earlier.

From that day on, Lena was committed to maintaining her healthy lifestyle. She knew that it wasn't just about looking good on the outside, but feeling good on the inside too. Lena had finally found the key to achieving her dream body, and she wasn't going to let it go.

The Beach Body Diet is a popular nutrition and fitness program designed to help individuals achieve a lean, toned physique that is ready for the beach. This diet emphasizes healthy eating habits, regular exercise, and lifestyle changes to promote overall health and wellness.

Many people turn to the Beach Body Diet as a way to lose weight, build muscle, and improve their overall fitness level.

The diet focuses on consuming whole, nutrient-dense foods, while limiting processed and sugary foods.

It also encourages regular exercise, such as strength training and cardiovascular activities, to promote muscle growth and weight loss.

One of the key principles of the Beach Body Diet is portion control. The diet emphasizes eating smaller, more frequent meals throughout the day, rather than relying on large, infrequent meals. Overeating is avoided and blood sugar levels are kept steady as a result.

Another important aspect of the Beach Body Diet is the emphasis on hydration. Drinking plenty of water is essential for optimal health, and it can help to flush toxins out of the body and promote healthy digestion.

The Beach Body Diet is not a quick-fix or fad diet, but rather a lifestyle change that encourages sustainable habits for long-term health and wellness. It emphasizes a balanced approach to eating and exercise, and encourages individuals to find the right balance that works for their unique needs and goals.

Overall, the Beach Body Diet is a comprehensive program that can help individuals achieve a healthy, toned physique that is ready for the beach. By focusing on healthy eating habits, regular exercise, and lifestyle changes, this program can help individuals achieve their goals and improve their overall health and well-being.

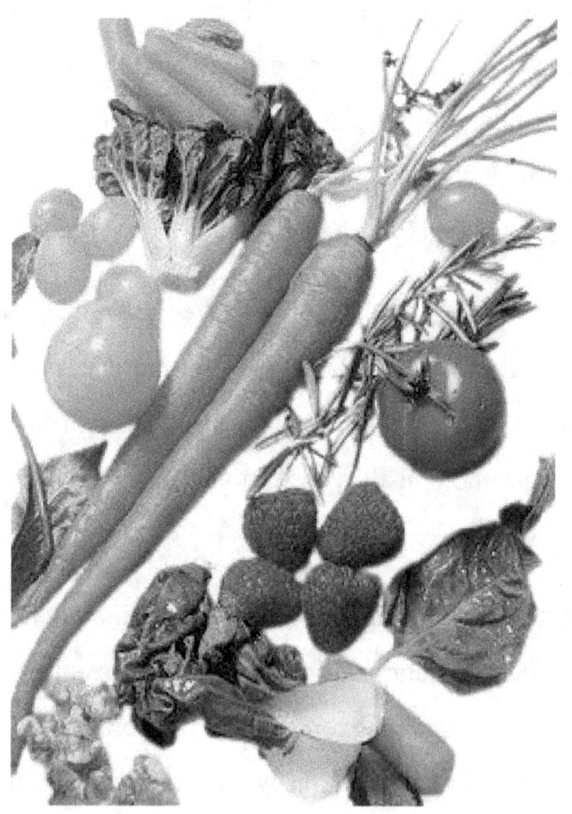

CHAPTER ONE

The Beach Body Diet Explained

The beach body diet is a popular eating plan that is designed to help people achieve a lean, toned body in time for summer.

This diet is often used by fitness enthusiasts, bodybuilders, and athletes to get in shape and achieve their fitness goals.

However, the beach body diet is not just for athletes; anyone who wants to lose weight and look great can benefit from following this diet plan.

The beach body diet is all about clean eating, which means avoiding processed foods and consuming whole, nutrient-dense foods instead.

This includes a variety of fruits and vegetables, lean proteins, complex carbohydrates, and healthy fats.

By focusing on these types of foods, you'll be able to provide your body with the nutrients it needs to build lean muscle, burn fat, and maintain a healthy weight.

One of the key principles of the beach body diet is to eat frequent, small meals throughout the day. This helps to keep your metabolism revved up, which means your body will burn more calories throughout the day.

Ideally, you should aim to eat 5-6 small meals per day, with each meal consisting of a lean protein source (such as chicken, fish, or tofu), complex carbohydrates (such as brown rice, quinoa, or sweet potato), and healthy fats (such as avocado, nuts, or olive oil).

In addition to eating clean, whole foods, the beach body diet also encourages you to drink plenty of water throughout the day. Staying hydrated is important for maintaining a healthy metabolism and helping your body flush out toxins.

Aim to drink at least 8 glasses of water per day, and more if you're exercising or spending time in the sun.

Another important component of the beach body diet is exercise. While you can certainly achieve a lean, toned body through diet alone, incorporating regular exercise into your routine can help you achieve your goals more quickly.

Ideally, you should aim to exercise for at least 30 minutes per day, five days per week. This can include a combination of cardio (such as running or cycling) and strength training (such as lifting weights or doing bodyweight exercises).

When it comes to snacks and treats, the beach body diet is all about balance. While it's important to avoid processed foods and sugary snacks, it's also important to give yourself a little bit of flexibility so you don't feel deprived. One way to do this is to allow yourself a cheat meal or two each week, where you can indulge in your favourite foods without worrying about sticking to your diet plan.

Overall, the beach body diet is a great way to achieve a lean, toned body in time for summer. By focusing on clean, whole foods and incorporating regular exercise into your routine, you'll be able to achieve your goals and look and feel your best. Yet, it's crucial to keep in mind that every person's body is unique, so what works for one person could not work for another. If you're not sure where to start, consider working with a registered dietitian or certified personal trainer to develop a customized plan that's tailored to your specific needs and goals.

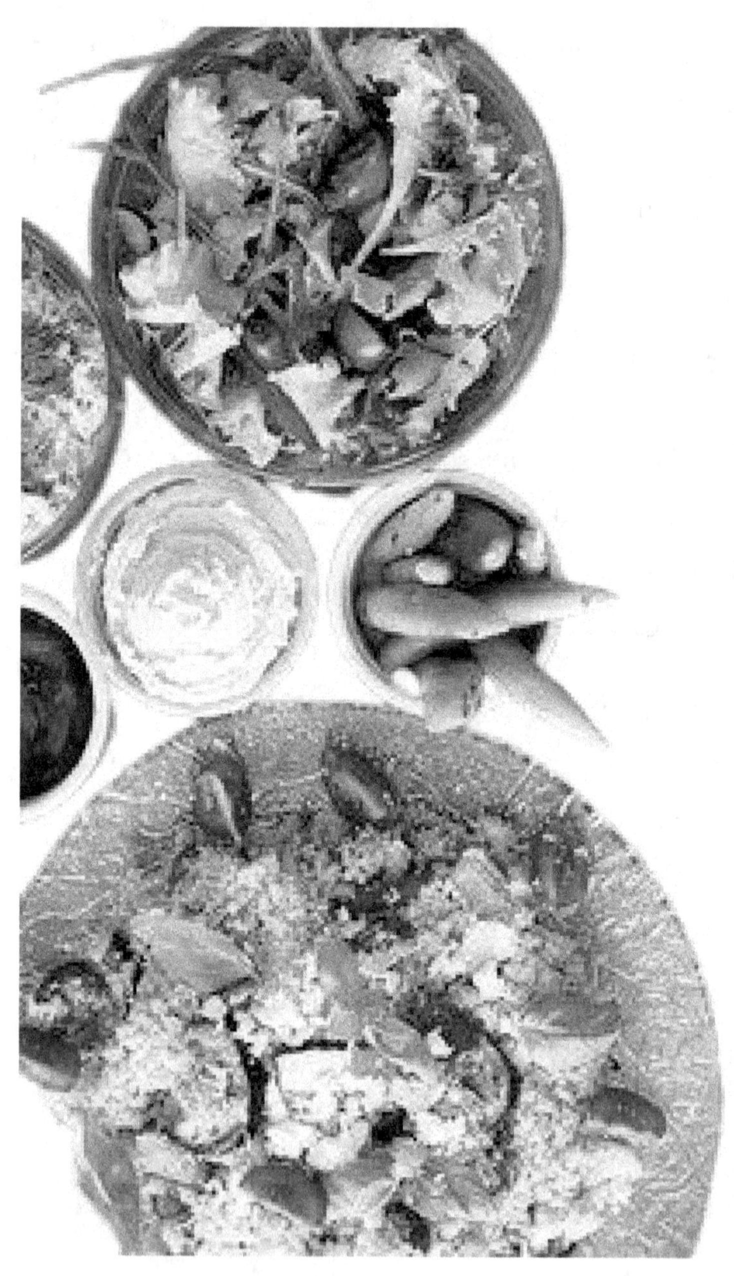

CHAPTER TWO

The Beach Body Diet and Benefits

The beach body diet is a term used to describe a diet and lifestyle regimen that aims to help individuals achieve a toned and fit physique in time for summer, beach season, or any other occasion where they may be exposing more skin.

This diet typically involves consuming nutrient-dense foods that are low in calories and high in fibre, protein, and healthy fats, while avoiding processed and high-sugar foods.

Benefits of the Beach Body Diet:

1. Weight Loss

One of the primary benefits of the beach body diet is weight loss. By consuming nutrient-dense, low-calorie foods, individuals can create a calorie deficit, which is essential for weight loss.

The diet also encourages the consumption of fibre-rich foods, which helps individuals feel fuller for longer, reducing the likelihood of overeating.

2. Improved Nutrient Intake

The beach body diet focuses on consuming nutrient-dense foods, which are high in vitamins and minerals that the body needs to function properly. By consuming a variety of fruits, vegetables, whole grains, lean proteins, and healthy fats, individuals can improve their overall nutrient intake and support their overall health and wellness.

3. Increased Energy Levels

Eating a healthy, balanced diet is essential for maintaining energy levels throughout the day. The beach body diet encourages the consumption of complex carbohydrates, which provide sustained energy, and protein, which helps to regulate blood sugar levels and prevent energy crashes.

4. Improved Digestive Health

The beach body diet is high in fibre, which is essential for digestive health. Fibre helps to regulate bowel movements and promotes the growth of healthy gut bacteria, which can improve overall digestive function and reduce the risk of digestive issues such as constipation and bloating.

5. Reduced Inflammation

The beach body diet emphasizes the consumption of anti-inflammatory foods, such as fruits, vegetables, whole grains, and healthy fats. These foods are high in antioxidants, which can help to reduce inflammation throughout the body and reduce the risk of chronic diseases such as heart disease, diabetes, and cancer.

6. Better Skin Health

Eating a healthy, balanced diet can also improve skin health. The beach body diet encourages the consumption of nutrient-dense foods that are high in vitamins, minerals, and antioxidants, which can help to improve skin elasticity, reduce inflammation, and protect against sun damage.

Tips for Following the Beach Body Diet

1. Focus on Whole, Nutrient-Dense Foods

To get the most out of the beach body diet, it is essential to focus on consuming whole, nutrient-dense foods such as fruits, vegetables, whole grains, lean proteins, and healthy fats. These foods are high in fibre, vitamins, and minerals and are essential for overall health and wellness.

2. Avoid Processed and High-Sugar Foods

To achieve a beach body, it is essential to avoid processed and high-sugar foods such as candy, soda, chips, and baked goods. These foods are typically high in calories, low in nutrients, and can contribute to weight gain and other health issues.

3. Stay Hydrated

Staying hydrated is essential for overall health and wellness, and it can also help to support weight loss. Drinking plenty of water can help individuals feel fuller for longer, reduce the likelihood of overeating, and improve overall digestive function.

4. Get Enough Sleep

Getting enough sleep is essential for overall health and wellness, and it can also support weight loss. Hormones that control hunger and fullness can be disturbed by sleep deprivation, which can result in overeating and weight gain.

5. Incorporate Exercise

While diet is essential for achieving a beach body, exercise is also crucial. Incorporating regular exercise, such as strength training and cardio, can help individuals build muscle and burn fat, leading to a toned and fit physique.

How to Follow the Beach Body Diet

A beach body diet is a specific diet that aims to help you achieve a toned and slim body, just in time for your next beach vacation.

It involves a combination of healthy eating habits and regular exercise to help you lose excess body fat and build lean muscle mass.

If you're looking to follow a beach body diet, here are some tips to get you started.

1. Set realistic goals:

Before you start any diet plan, it's essential to set realistic goals. You don't want to aim for a weight loss target that's unachievable, as this can lead to disappointment and frustration.

Instead, aim to lose a pound or two each week, which is a healthy and sustainable rate of weight loss. This way, you'll be more likely to stick to your diet plan and see results.

2. Incorporate lean protein:

Protein is a necessary nutrient that is important for the growth and repair of muscular tissue. As part of your beach body diet, aim to incorporate lean protein sources such as chicken, turkey, fish, tofu, and legumes into your meals. These foods will keep you feeling fuller for longer and help you maintain your energy levels throughout the day.

3. Increase your vegetable intake:

Vegetables are packed with essential vitamins, minerals, and antioxidants that are crucial for overall health and wellbeing. As part of your beach body diet, aim to increase your vegetable intake by adding a variety of colourful veggies to your meals. Some great options include broccoli, spinach, kale, sweet potato, and carrots.

4. Limit processed foods:

Processed foods such as chips, crackers, and sugary snacks are often high in calories, unhealthy fats, and added sugars.

As part of your beach body diet, aim to limit your intake of these foods and replace them with healthier alternatives such as fruits, nuts, and whole-grain crackers.

5. Drink plenty of water:

Staying hydrated is crucial for maintaining good health and helping to flush toxins from your body. As part of your beach body diet, aim to drink at least eight glasses of water each day. You can also add lemon or lime to your water to add flavour and help with digestion.

6. Incorporate healthy fats:

Healthy fats such as avocado, nuts, and olive oil are essential for maintaining good health and supporting your body's natural processes. As part of your beach body diet, aim to incorporate healthy fats into your meals to help you feel fuller for longer and maintain your energy levels.

7. Exercise regularly:

Regular exercise is a key component of any beach body diet plan. Try to do moderate-intensity activity for at least 30 minutes each day, such as brisk walking, cycling, or swimming. You can also incorporate strength training exercises such as weightlifting or resistance band workouts to help build lean muscle mass and improve your overall fitness levels.

7 Day Beach Body Diet Meal Plan

Day 1

Breakfast:

Greek Yogurt with Berries and Almonds

Ingredients:

- 1 cup plain Greek yogurt

- 1/2 cup mixed berries

- 1/4 cup sliced almonds

Preparation:

1. In a bowl, combine Greek yogurt, mixed berries, and sliced almonds.

2. Serve and enjoy.

Snack:

Apple slices with Almond Butter

Ingredients:

- 1 medium apple, sliced

- 2 tbsp almond butter

Preparation:

1. Spread almond butter on apple slices.

2. Serve and enjoy.

Lunch:

Grilled Chicken Salad

Ingredients:

- 4 oz grilled chicken breast

- 2 cups mixed greens

- 1/2 cup cherry tomatoes

- 1/4 cup sliced cucumbers

- 1/4 cup sliced red onions

- 1 tbsp balsamic vinaigrette

Preparation:

1. In a large bowl, combine mixed greens, cherry tomatoes, sliced cucumbers, and sliced red onions.

2. Top with grilled chicken breast.

3. Drizzle balsamic vinaigrette over the salad.

4. Serve and enjoy.

Snack:

Carrot Sticks with Hummus

Ingredients:

- 1 cup carrot sticks

- 2 tbsp hummus

Preparation:

1. Serve carrot sticks with hummus for dipping.

2. Serve and enjoy.

Dinner:

Baked Cod with Quinoa and Asparagus

Ingredients:

- 4 oz cod fillet

- 1/2 cup quinoa

- 1/2 cup asparagus spears

- 1/2 tbsp olive oil

- 1/4 tsp salt

- 1/4 tsp black pepper

Preparation:

1. Preheat oven to 400°F (200°C).

2. Season cod fillet with salt and black pepper.

3. Place cod fillet on a baking sheet and bake for 12-15 minutes or until fully cooked.

4. In a separate pot, cook quinoa according to package instructions.

5. Olive oil should be heated to a medium-high haze in a big skillet.

6. Add asparagus spears and cook for 5-7 minutes or until tender.

7. Serve baked cod with quinoa and asparagus.

8. Enjoy.

Day 2

Breakfast:

Veggie Omelette

Ingredients:

- 2 eggs

- 1/4 cup chopped spinach

- 1/4 cup chopped bell peppers

- 1/4 cup chopped onions

- 1/4 cup shredded cheddar cheese

- 1 tsp olive oil

Preparation:

1. Beat eggs with a fork in a bowl.

2. Over medium-high heat, warm up the olive oil in a big skillet.

3. Add chopped spinach, bell peppers, and onions to the skillet.

4. Cook vegetables until tender, stirring occasionally.

5. Pour beaten eggs over the cooked vegetables in the skillet.

6. Sprinkle shredded cheddar cheese over the omelette.

7. To fold the omelette in half, use a spatula.

8. Cook until the cheese is melted and the eggs are fully cooked.

9. Serve and enjoy.

Snack:

Cottage Cheese with Pineapple

Ingredients:

- 1/2 cup low-fat cottage cheese

- 1/2 cup chopped pineapple

Preparation:

1. In a bowl, combine low-fat cottage cheese and chopped pineapple.

2. Serve and enjoy.

Lunch:

Tuna Salad with Crackers

Ingredients:

- 1 can tuna in water, drained

- 1/4 cup chopped celery

- 1/4 cup chopped red onions

- 1 tbsp mayonnaise

- 1 tbsp lemon juice

- Salt and black pepper, to taste

Whole grain crackers

Preparation:

1. In a bowl, combine drained tuna, chopped celery, and chopped red onions.

2. Add mayonnaise and lemon juice to the bowl and mix well.

3. To taste, add salt and black pepper to the dish.

4. Serve tuna salad with whole grain crackers.

5. Enjoy.

Snack:

Banana Smoothie

Ingredients:

- 1 ripe banana

- 1/2 cup unsweetened almond milk

- 1/2 cup plain Greek yogurt

- 1 tsp honey

- 1/4 tsp vanilla extract

- 1/2 cup ice

Preparation:

1. Add banana, almond milk, Greek yogurt, honey, vanilla extract, and ice to a blender.

2. Blend until smooth.

3. Serve and enjoy.

Dinner:

Grilled Shrimp with Zucchini Noodles

Ingredients:

- 4 oz shrimp, peeled and deveined

- 1 medium zucchini, spiralized

- 1/4 cup cherry tomatoes

- 1 tbsp olive oil

- 1 garlic clove, minced

- Salt and black pepper, to taste

Preparation:

1. Preheat grill to medium-high heat.

2. In a bowl, combine shrimp, olive oil, minced garlic, salt, and black pepper.

3. Thread shrimp onto skewers and grill for 2-3 minutes per side or until fully cooked.

4. Olive oil should be heated in a different pan over medium-high heat.

5. Add spiralized zucchini noodles and cherry tomatoes to the pan.

6. Cook for 2-3 minutes or until zucchini noodles are tender.

7. Serve grilled shrimp with zucchini noodles.

8. Enjoy.

Day 3

Breakfast:

Blueberry Smoothie Bowl

Ingredients:

- 1/2 cup frozen blueberries

- 1/2 banana

- 1/2 cup unsweetened almond milk

- 1/4 cup rolled oats

- 1 tbsp almond butter

- 1 tbsp honey

- 1/4 tsp vanilla extract

Toppings:

- Sliced banana

- Sliced almonds

- Chia seeds

Preparation:

1. Add frozen blueberries, banana, almond milk, rolled oats, almond butter, honey, and vanilla extract to a blender.

2. Blend until smooth and creamy.

3. Pour smoothie into a bowl.

4. Top with sliced banana, sliced almonds, and chia seeds.

5. Enjoy.

Snack:

Cherry Tomatoes with Mozzarella Cheese

Ingredients:

- 1 cup cherry tomatoes

- 1 oz mozzarella cheese, cubed

Preparation:

1. In a bowl, combine cherry tomatoes and cubed mozzarella cheese.

2. Serve and enjoy.

Lunch:

Grilled Chicken Wrap

Ingredients:

- 4 oz grilled chicken breast, sliced

- 1 large whole wheat tortilla

- 1/4 cup sliced avocado

- 1/4 cup shredded lettuce

- 1/4 cup sliced red onions

- 1 tbsp Greek yogurt

- 1 tbsp salsa

Preparation:

1. Place sliced grilled chicken breast on a whole wheat tortilla.

2. Top with sliced avocado, shredded lettuce, and sliced red onions.

3. Drizzle Greek yogurt and salsa over the ingredients.

4. Slice the tortilla in half after rolling it up.

5. Serve and enjoy.

Snack:

Chocolate Protein Shake

Ingredients:

- 1 scoop chocolate protein powder

- 1/2 banana

- 1 cup unsweetened almond milk

- 1/2 cup ice

Preparation:

1. Add chocolate protein powder, banana, almond milk, and ice to a blender.

2. Blend until smooth and creamy.

3. Serve and enjoy.

Dinner:

Lemon Herb Salmon with Roasted Asparagus

Ingredients:

- 4 oz salmon fillet

- 1 lemon, sliced

- 1 tbsp chopped fresh parsley

- 1 tbsp chopped fresh dill

- 1 garlic clove, minced

- Salt and black pepper, to taste

- 1 lb asparagus

- 1 tbsp olive oil

- Salt and black pepper, to taste

Preparation:

1. Preheat oven to 400°F.

2. Season salmon fillet with salt and black pepper on both sides.

3. Place salmon fillet in a baking dish and top with lemon slices, chopped fresh parsley, chopped fresh dill, and minced garlic.

4. Bake salmon for 12-15 minutes or until fully cooked.

5. In a separate baking dish, toss asparagus with olive oil, salt, and black pepper.

6. Roast asparagus for 12-15 minutes or until tender.

7. Serve lemon herb salmon with roasted asparagus.

8. Enjoy.

Day 4

Breakfast:

Greek Yogurt with Mixed Berries and Granola

Ingredients:

- 1/2 cup plain Greek yogurt

- a half-cup of mixed berries (such as raspberries, blueberries, and strawberries)

- 1/4 cup granola

Preparation:

- In a bowl, mix together Greek yogurt and mixed berries.

- Top with granola.

- Enjoy.

Snack:

Apple Slices with Peanut Butter

Ingredients:

- 1 apple, sliced

- 1 tbsp natural peanut butter

Preparation:

1. Spread peanut butter over apple slices.

2. Serve and enjoy.

Lunch:

Tuna Avocado Salad

Ingredients:

- 1 can tuna, drained

- 1/2 avocado, diced

- 1/4 cup chopped red onions

- 1 tbsp mayonnaise

- 1 tbsp lemon juice

- Salt and black pepper, to taste

- Whole grain crackers

Preparation:

1. In a bowl, combine drained tuna, diced avocado, and chopped red onions.

2. Add mayonnaise and lemon juice to the bowl and mix well.

3. To taste, add salt and black pepper to the dish.

4. Serve tuna avocado salad with whole grain crackers.

5. Enjoy.

Snack:

Carrots and Hummus

Ingredients:

- 1 cup baby carrots

- 2 tbsp hummus

- Preparation:

- Serve baby carrots with hummus.

- Enjoy.

Dinner:

Chicken Fajita Bowl

Ingredients:

- 4 oz chicken breast, sliced

- 1/2 red bell pepper, sliced

- 1/2 yellow bell pepper, sliced

- 1/4 cup sliced red onions

- 1 tbsp olive oil

- 1 tsp chili powder

- 1/2 tsp cumin

- Salt and black pepper, to taste

- 1 cup cooked brown rice

- 1/4 cup shredded cheddar cheese

- 1/4 cup salsa

Preparation:

1. Olive oil should be heated in a pan over a medium heat.

2. Add sliced chicken breast, sliced red and yellow bell peppers, and sliced red onions to the pan.

3. Season with chili powder, cumin, salt, and black pepper.

4. Cook the chicken for an additional 5-7 minutes, or until done.

5. Serve cooked brown rice in a bowl.

6. Top with chicken and vegetables, shredded cheddar cheese, and salsa.

7. Enjoy.

Day 5

Breakfast:

Spinach and Feta Omelette

Ingredients:

- 2 eggs

- 1/4 cup baby spinach

- 1/4 cup crumbled feta cheese

- Salt and black pepper, to taste

- 1 tsp olive oil

Preparation:

1. In a bowl, beat eggs until fully mixed.

2. Add baby spinach, crumbled feta cheese, salt, and black pepper to the bowl and mix well.

3. Over medium heat, warm the olive oil in the pan.

4. Pour egg mixture into the pan and cook for 2-3 minutes or until the bottom is set.

5. Fold the omelette in half using a spatula.

6. Cook for a further 1-2 minutes, or until done.

7. Serve and enjoy.

Snack:

Protein Smoothie

Ingredients:

*   1 scoop vanilla protein powder

*   1/2 banana

*   1/2 cup unsweetened almond milk

*   1/2 cup frozen mixed berries

Preparation:

1. Add all ingredients to a blender.

2. Blend until smooth and creamy.

3. Serve and enjoy.

Lunch:

Shrimp and Quinoa Salad

Ingredients:

- 4 oz cooked shrimp

- 1 cup cooked quinoa

- 1/2 avocado, diced

- 1/4 cup cherry tomatoes, halved

- 1 tbsp chopped fresh cilantro

- 1 tbsp olive oil

- 1 tbsp lime juice

- Salt and black pepper, to taste

Preparation:

1. In a bowl, combine cooked shrimp, cooked quinoa, diced avocado, cherry tomatoes, and chopped fresh cilantro.

2. In a separate bowl, whisk together olive oil, lime juice, salt, and black pepper.

3. Mix the salad thoroughly after adding the dressing.

4. Serve and enjoy.

Snack:

Cottage Cheese with Pineapple

Ingredients:

- 1/2 cup low-fat cottage cheese

- 1/2 cup fresh pineapple chunks

Preparation:

1. In a bowl, mix together low-fat cottage cheese and fresh pineapple chunks.

2. Serve and enjoy.

Dinner:

Grilled Chicken with Zucchini and Squash

Ingredients:

- 4 oz chicken breast

- 1 small zucchini, sliced

- 1 small yellow squash, sliced

- 1 tbsp olive oil

- Salt and black pepper, to taste

Preparation:

1. Preheat grill to medium-high heat.

2. Season chicken breast with salt and black pepper on both sides.

3. Brush zucchini and squash slices with olive oil and season with salt and black pepper.

4. Grill chicken breast for 5-7 minutes on each side or until fully cooked.

5. Grill zucchini and squash slices for 3-4 minutes on each side or until tender.

6. Serve grilled chicken breast with grilled zucchini and squash slices.

7. Enjoy.

Day 6

Breakfast:

Overnight Oats with Berries and Almonds

Ingredients:

- 1/2 cup rolled oats

- 1/2 cup unsweetened almond milk

- a half-cup of mixed berries (such as raspberries, blueberries, and strawberries)

- 1 tbsp sliced almonds

- 1 tsp honey

Preparation:

1. In a jar or bowl, mix together rolled oats and unsweetened almond milk.

2. Cover and refrigerate overnight.

3. In the morning, top with mixed berries, sliced almonds, and honey.

4. Serve and enjoy.

Snack:

Hard-Boiled Egg with Tomato Slices

Ingredients:

- 1 hard-boiled egg

- 1 medium tomato, sliced

Preparation:

1. Serve hard-boiled egg with tomato slices.

2. Enjoy.

Lunch:

Turkey and Cheese Wrap

Ingredients:

- 2 slices of low-sodium turkey breast

- 1 slice of low-fat cheese

- 1 whole wheat tortilla

- 1/4 avocado, mashed

- 1/4 cup baby spinach

- 1 tbsp Dijon mustard

Preparation:

1. On a plate or cutting board, place the whole-wheat tortilla flat.

2. Spread mashed avocado over the tortilla.

3. Place turkey slices, cheese slice, and baby spinach on top of the avocado.

4. Drizzle Dijon mustard over the filling.

5. Slice the tortilla in half after tightly rolling it.

6. Serve and enjoy.

Snack:

Apple Slices with Peanut Butter

Ingredients:

- 1 medium apple, sliced

- 1 tbsp natural peanut butter

Preparation:

1. Spread natural peanut butter over apple slices.

2. Serve and enjoy.

Dinner:

Brown rice, asparagus, and baked salmon

Ingredients:

- 4 oz salmon fillet

- 1/2 bunch asparagus, trimmed

- 1/2 cup brown rice

- 1 tbsp olive oil

- Salt and black pepper, to taste

- 1/2 lemon, sliced

Preparation:

1. Preheat oven to 375°F.

2. Cook brown rice according to package instructions.

3. In a baking dish, place salmon fillet and asparagus.

4. Olive oil should be drizzled over the salmon and asparagus.

5. Season with salt and black pepper.

6. Slices of lemon should be placed above the fish.

7. Salmon should be baked for 15 to 20 minutes, or until done.

8. Serve baked salmon and asparagus with brown rice.

9. Enjoy.

Day 7

Breakfast:

Greek Yogurt with Granola and Berries

Ingredients:

- 1/2 cup non-fat Greek yogurt

- 1/4 cup granola

- 1/4 cup mixed berries (such as raspberries, blueberries, and strawberries)

Preparation:

1. In a bowl, mix together non-fat Greek yogurt and granola.

2. Top with mixed berries.

3. Serve and enjoy.

Snack:

Carrot Sticks with Hummus

Ingredients:

- 1 medium carrot, sliced into sticks

- 2 tbsp hummus

Preparation:

1. Dip carrot sticks in hummus.

2. Serve and enjoy.

Lunch:

Tuna Salad Lettuce Wraps

Ingredients:

- 1 can of tuna, drained

- 1/4 cup chopped celery

- 1/4 cup chopped red onion

- 1 tbsp lemon juice

- 1 tbsp olive oil

- Salt and black pepper, to taste

- 4 large lettuce leaves

Preparation:

1. In a bowl, mix together drained tuna, chopped celery, chopped red onion, lemon juice, olive oil, salt, and black pepper.

2. Lay lettuce leaves flat on a plate or cutting board.

3. Place tuna salad on top of the lettuce leaves.

4. Roll the lettuce leaves tightly to form wraps.

5. Serve and enjoy.

Snack:

Mixed Nuts and Seeds

Ingredients:

- 1/4 cup mixed nuts (such as almonds, cashews, and pistachios)

- 1 tbsp mixed seeds (such as pumpkin seeds and sunflower seeds)

Preparation:

1. Mix together mixed nuts and seeds.

2. Serve and enjoy.

Dinner:

Grilled Shrimp Skewers with Pineapple and Bell Pepper

Ingredients:

- 4 oz raw shrimp, peeled and deveined

- 1/2 cup fresh pineapple chunks

- 1/2 red bell pepper, sliced into pieces

- 1/2 yellow bell pepper, sliced into pieces

- 1 tbsp olive oil

- Salt and black pepper, to taste

- 2 wooden skewers

Preparation:

1. Preheat grill to medium-high heat.

2. For ten to fifteen minutes, soak wooden skewers in water.

3. Thread shrimp, pineapple chunks, and bell pepper
    pieces onto the skewers.

4. Brush olive oil over the skewers.

5. Season with salt and black pepper.

6. Place skewers on the grill and cook for 3-4 minutes
    on each side, or until shrimp is fully cooked.

7. Serve grilled shrimp skewers with a side salad.

8. Enjoy.

Snack:

Greek Yogurt with Cinnamon and Honey

Ingredients:

- 1/2 cup non-fat Greek yogurt

- 1/4 tsp cinnamon

- 1 tbsp honey

Preparation:

1. In a bowl, mix together non-fat Greek yogurt, cinnamon, and honey.

2. Serve and enjoy.

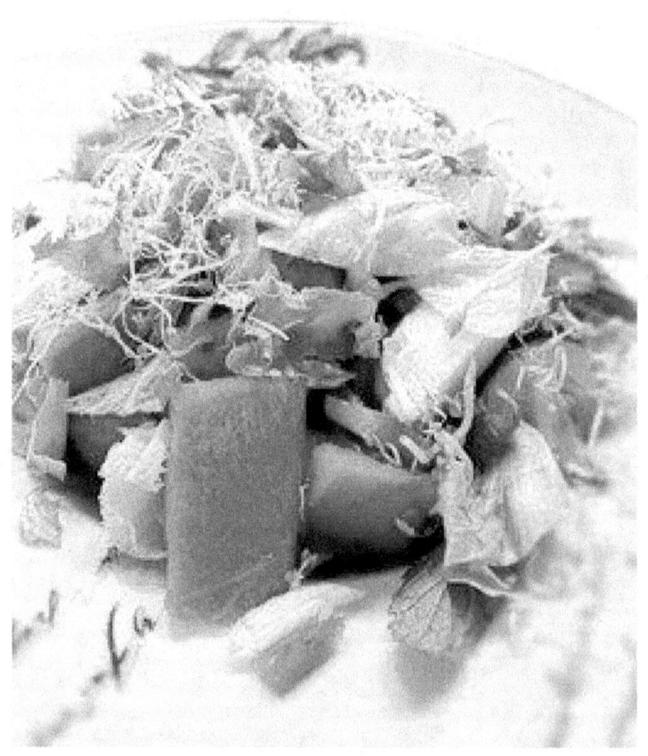

CHAPTER THREE

The Beach Body Diet Recipes

1. Grilled Shrimp Skewers:

This protein-packed dish is perfect for a light lunch or dinner on the beach.

Ingredients:

- 1 pound of peeled and deveined big shrimp

- 1/4 cup of olive oil

- 2 tablespoons of minced garlic

- Salt and pepper

- Lemon wedges

Instructions:

1. Preheat the grill to medium-high heat.

2. Thread the shrimp onto skewers.

3. Mix the olive oil, garlic, salt, and pepper in a small bowl.

4. Brush the mixture over the shrimp skewers.

5. Grill the shrimp for 2-3 minutes on each side, until they are pink and cooked through.

6. Serve with lemon wedges.

Cooking Time: 10 minutes

2. Quinoa Salad:

This refreshing salad is packed with nutrients and perfect for a beach picnic.

Ingredients:

- 1 cup of cooked quinoa

- 1/2 cup of chopped cucumber

- 1/2 cup of chopped cherry tomatoes

- 1/4 cup of chopped red onion

- 1/4 cup of chopped fresh parsley

- 2 tablespoons of olive oil

- 1 tablespoon of lemon juice

- Salt and pepper

Instructions:

1. In a large bowl, combine the cooked quinoa, cucumber, cherry tomatoes, red onion, and parsley.

2. Mix the olive oil, lemon juice, salt, and pepper in a small bowl.

3. After adding the dressing, toss the salad to incorporate.

4. Serve chilled.

Cooking Time: 15 minutes

3. Grilled Salmon with Avocado Salsa:

This flavourful dish is full of healthy fats and perfect for a beachside dinner.

Ingredients:

- 4 salmon fillets

- Salt and pepper

- 2 avocados, diced

- 1/4 cup of chopped red onion

- 1/4 cup of chopped cilantro

- 1 jalapeno pepper, seeded and minced

- 2 tablespoons of lime juice

- 2 tablespoons of olive oil

Instructions:

1. Preheat the grill to medium-high heat.

2. Add salt and pepper to the salmon fillets.

3. In a small bowl, combine the diced avocado, red onion, cilantro, jalapeno pepper, lime juice, and olive oil.

4. The salmon fillets should be cooked through after grilling for 4–5 minutes on each side.

5. Serve the salmon topped with the salsa made from avocados.

Cooking Time: 20 minutes

4. Greek Yogurt Parfait:

This easy and healthy breakfast is perfect for a day at the beach.

Ingredients:

- 1 cup of Greek yogurt

- 1/2 cup of fresh berries

- 1/4 cup of granola

- 1 tablespoon of honey

Instructions:

1. In a glass or jar, layer the Greek yogurt, fresh berries, and granola.

2. Drizzle the honey on top.

3. Serve immediately.

Cooking Time: 5 minutes

5. Tuna Salad Lettuce Wraps:

These low-carb wraps are perfect for a light lunch on the beach.

Ingredients:

- 2 cans of tuna, drained

- 1/4 cup of chopped celery

- 1/4 cup of chopped red onion

- 1/4 cup of chopped dill pickles

- 2 tablespoons of olive oil

- 2 tablespoons of lemon juice

- Salt and pepper

- Lettuce leaves

Instructions:

1. In a large bowl, combine the tuna, celery, red onion, and dill pickles.

2. Mix the olive oil, lemon juice, salt, and pepper in a small bowl.

3. After adding the dressing, whisk the tuna mixture to incorporate.

4. Spoon the tuna salad onto lettuce leaves and wrap them up.

5. Serve immediately.

Cooking Time: 10 minutes

6. Veggie Burger:

This plant-based burger is a healthier alternative to a traditional burger and perfect for a beach picnic.

Ingredients:

- Drained and washed black beans from one can

- 1/2 cup of cooked quinoa

- 1/4 cup of chopped red onion

- 1/4 cup of chopped bell pepper

- 2 tablespoons of chopped cilantro

- 1 teaspoon of cumin

- 1 teaspoon of chili powder

- Salt and pepper

- Whole wheat burger buns

- selection of toppings (lettuce, tomato, avocado, etc.)

Instructions:

1. Using a fork, mash the black beans in a big bowl.

2. Add the cooked quinoa, red onion, bell pepper, cilantro, cumin, chili powder, salt, and pepper. Stir to combine.

3. Form the mixture into patties.

4. Grill or grill pan should be heated to medium-high.

5. Grill the veggie burgers for 3-4 minutes on each side, until they are browned and heated through.

6. Serve the burgers on whole wheat buns with your favourite toppings.

Cooking Time: 25 minutes

7. Watermelon Salad:

This refreshing salad is perfect for a hot day on the beach.

Ingredients:

- 4 cups of cubed watermelon

- 1/2 cup of crumbled feta cheese

- 1/4 cup of chopped fresh mint

- 2 tablespoons of olive oil

- 2 tablespoons of balsamic vinegar

- Salt and pepper

Instructions:

1. In a large bowl, combine the cubed watermelon, crumbled feta cheese, and chopped mint.

2. Mix the olive oil, balsamic vinegar, salt, and pepper in a small basin.

3. Mix the watermelon mixture with the dressing after pouring it over it.

4. Serve chilled.

Cooking Time: 10 minutes

8. Grilled Chicken Salad:

This protein-packed salad is perfect for a beachside lunch.

Ingredients:

- 2 chicken breasts

- Salt and pepper

- 4 cups of mixed greens

- 1/2 cup of cherry tomatoes

- 1/4 cup of chopped red onion

- 1/4 cup of chopped cucumber

- 2 tablespoons of olive oil

- 2 tablespoons of lemon juice

Instructions:

1. Preheat the grill to medium-high heat.

2. Chicken breasts should be salted and peppered.

3. Grill the chicken for 5-6 minutes on each side, until they are cooked through.

4. Let the chicken rest for 5 minutes, then slice it.

5. The mixed greens, cherry tomatoes, red onion, and cucumber should all be combined in a big bowl.

6. Mix the olive oil, lemon juice, salt, and pepper in a small bowl.

7. After adding the dressing, toss the salad to incorporate.

8. Top the salad with the sliced chicken.

Cooking Time: 25 minutes

9. Grilled Zucchini:

This simple side dish is a delicious way to get your veggies in on the beach.

Ingredients:

- 2 zucchinis, sliced lengthwise

- 2 tablespoons of olive oil

- Salt and pepper

Instructions:

1. Preheat the grill to medium-high heat.

2. Salt and pepper the zucchini slices after brushing
    them with olive oil.

3. Grill the zucchini for 3-4 minutes on each side, until
    they are tender and grill marks appear.

4. Serve hot.

Cooking Time: 10 minutes

10. Greek Yogurt Parfait:

This light and healthy dessert is perfect for a beach day.

Ingredients:

- 1 cup of plain Greek yogurt

- 1/4 cup of granola

- 1/4 cup of sliced strawberries

- 1/4 cup of blueberries

- 1 tablespoon of honey

Instructions:

1. In a small glass or jar, layer the Greek yogurt, granola, sliced strawberries, and blueberries.

2. Drizzle honey over the top.

3. Serve chilled.

Cooking Time: 5 minutes

11. Grilled Shrimp Skewers:

These skewers are a delicious and easy way to enjoy seafood on the beach.

Ingredients:

- 1 pound of peeled and deveined big shrimp

- 2 tablespoons of olive oil

- 2 tablespoons of lemon juice

- 2 cloves of garlic, minced

- Salt and pepper

- 30-minute-soaked wooden skewers in water

Instructions:

1. Preheat the grill to medium-high heat.

2. Mix the olive oil, lemon juice, garlic, salt, and pepper in a sizable bowl.

3. The shrimp should be added to the bowl and coated.

4. Thread the shrimp onto the skewers.

5. Grill the shrimp skewers for 2-3 minutes on each side, until they are pink and opaque.

6. Serve hot.

Cooking Time: 15 minutes

12. Quinoa Salad:

This protein-packed salad is perfect for a healthy beach picnic.

Ingredients:

- 1 cup of cooked quinoa

- 1/2 cup of chopped cucumber

- 1/2 cup of cherry tomatoes, halved

- 1/4 cup of chopped red onion

- 1/4 cup of chopped fresh parsley

- 2 tablespoons of olive oil

- 2 tablespoons of lemon juice

- Salt and pepper

Instructions:

1. In a large bowl, combine the cooked quinoa, chopped cucumber, cherry tomatoes, red onion, and parsley.

2. Mix the olive oil, lemon juice, salt, and pepper in a small bowl.

3. Toss the quinoa mixture with the dressing after pouring it over it.

4. Serve chilled.

Cooking Time: 15 minutes

13. Grilled Fish Tacos:

These tacos are a fun and delicious way to enjoy fish on the beach.

Ingredients:

- 1 pound of white fish (such as cod or halibut)

- 1 tablespoon of olive oil

- 1 tablespoon of chili powder

- 1/2 teaspoon of garlic powder

- Salt and pepper

- Corn tortillas

Toppings of your choice (shredded cabbage, sliced avocado, chopped cilantro, lime wedges, etc.)

Instructions:

1. Preheat the grill to medium-high heat.

2. In a small bowl, whisk together the olive oil, chili powder, garlic powder, salt, and pepper.

3. Brush the fish with the spice mixture.

4. Grill the fish for 3-4 minutes on each side, until it is cooked through.

5. Heat the corn tortillas on the grill for 30 seconds on each side.

6. Flake the fish into pieces.

7. Assemble the tacos with the fish and your favourite toppings.

Cooking Time: 20 minutes

14. Berry Smoothie:

This refreshing smoothie is perfect for a hot day on the beach.

Ingredients:

- 1 cup of mixed frozen berries

- 1 banana

- 1/2 cup of Greek yogurt

- 1/2 cup of almond milk

- 1 tablespoon of honey

- Ice (optional)

Instructions:

1. Add the frozen berries, banana, Greek yogurt, almond milk, and honey to a blender.

2. Blend until smooth.

3. Add ice if desired and blend again.

4. Serve cold.

Cooking Time: 5 minutes

15. Grilled Chicken Skewers:

These chicken skewers are a classic beach dish that everyone will love.

Ingredients:

- 1 pound of cubed, skinless, boneless chicken breasts

- 2 tablespoons of olive oil

- 2 tablespoons of lemon juice

- 2 cloves of garlic, minced

- Salt and pepper

- 30-minute-soaked wooden skewers in water

Instructions:

1. Preheat the grill to medium-high heat.

2. Mix the olive oil, lemon juice, garlic, salt, and pepper in a sizable bowl.

3. The chicken should be added to the bowl and coated.

4. Thread the chicken onto the skewers.

5. Grill the chicken skewers for 5-6 minutes on each side, until they are cooked through.

6. Serve hot.

Cooking Time: 20 minutes

16. Summer Fruit Salad:

This colourful fruit salad is a refreshing and healthy option for the beach.

Ingredients:

- 2 cups of mixed fruit (such as strawberries, blueberries, raspberries, watermelon, and pineapple)

- 1 tablespoon of honey

- 1 tablespoon of lime juice

- 1 tablespoon of chopped fresh mint

Instructions:

1. Cut the fruit into bite-sized pieces and add them to a large bowl.

2. Mix the honey, lime juice, and mint in a small basin.

3. Toss the fruit with the dressing after pouring it over it.

4. Serve chilled.

Cooking Time: 10 minutes

17. Grilled Steak Salad:

This hearty salad is a great option for a beach lunch.

Ingredients:

- 1 pound of flank steak

- 1 tablespoon of olive oil

- Salt and pepper

- 6 cups of mixed greens

- 1/2 cup of cherry tomatoes, halved

- 1/2 cup of sliced cucumber

- 1/4 cup of chopped red onion

- 1/4 cup of crumbled feta cheese

- 2 tablespoons of balsamic vinegar

- 2 tablespoons of olive oil

Instructions:

1. Preheat the grill to medium-high heat.

2. Olive oil should be used to rub the meat before adding salt and pepper.

3. Grill the steak for 4-5 minutes on each side, until it is cooked to your liking.

4. Before slicing the steak thinly across the grain, give it five minutes to rest.

5. The mixed greens, cherry tomatoes, cucumber, red onion, and feta cheese should all be combined in a big bowl.

6. Combine the olive oil and balsamic vinegar in a small bowl.

7. Toss the salad with the dressing after pouring it over it.

8. Top the salad with the sliced steak.

9. Serve chilled.

Cooking Time: 25 minutes

18. Grilled Veggie Wraps:

These wraps are a healthy and satisfying lunch option for the beach.

Ingredients:

- 2 large zucchinis, sliced lengthwise

- 2 large bell peppers, sliced into strips

- 1 red onion, sliced into rings

- 2 tablespoons of olive oil

- Salt and pepper

- 4 whole wheat tortillas

- 1/2 cup of hummus

- 1/2 cup of crumbled feta cheese

Instructions:

1. Preheat the grill to medium-high heat.

2. In a large bowl, toss the zucchini, bell peppers, and red onion with olive oil, salt, and pepper.

3. Grill the veggies for 3-4 minutes on each side, until they are tender and slightly charred.

4. Grilling the tortillas for 30 seconds on each side will preheat them.

5. Spread each tortilla with a generous spoonful of hummus.

6. Add a few slices of grilled veggies to each tortilla.

7. Top the vegetables with feta cheese.

8. Roll up the tortillas and serve.

Cooking Time: 20 minutes

19. Quinoa and Black Bean Salad:

This protein-packed salad is a great option for a beach picnic.

Ingredients:

- 1 cup of quinoa

- 2 cups of water

- 1 can of rinsed and drained black beans

- 1 red bell pepper, chopped

- 1/2 red onion, chopped

- 1 avocado, diced

- 1/4 cup of chopped fresh cilantro

- 2 tablespoons of olive oil

- 2 tablespoons of lime juice

- Salt and pepper

Instructions:

1. Rinse the quinoa in a fine-mesh strainer.

2. Bring the water to a rolling boil in a medium saucepan.

3. Add the quinoa to the saucepan and reduce the heat to low.

4. Cover the saucepan and simmer for 15-20 minutes, until the quinoa is tender and the water is absorbed.

5. Combine the cooked quinoa, black beans, red onion, red bell pepper, avocado, and cilantro in a sizable bowl.

6. Mix the olive oil, lime juice, salt, and pepper in a small bowl.

7. Toss the salad with the dressing after pouring it over it.

8. Serve chilled.

Cooking Time: 25 minutes

20. Grilled Fish Tacos:

These fish tacos are a beach classic.

Ingredients:

- 1 pound of white fish fillets (such as tilapia or cod)

- 2 tablespoons of olive oil

- Salt and pepper

- 1/4 cup of plain Greek yogurt

- 1 tablespoon of lime juice

- 1/4 teaspoon of cumin

- 1/4 teaspoon of chili powder

- 8 corn tortillas

- 1/2 cup of shredded cabbage

- 1/2 cup of Pico de Gallo

Instructions:

1. Preheat the grill to medium-high heat.

2. Salt and pepper the fish fillets after rubbing them with olive oil.

3. Grill the fish for 3-4 minutes on each side, until it is cooked through.

4. Combine the Greek yogurt, lime juice, cumin, and chili powder in a small bowl.

5. Grilling the tortillas for 30 seconds on each side will preheat them.

6. To assemble the tacos, place a few pieces of grilled fish on each tortilla.

7. Top the fish with shredded cabbage and Pico de Gallo.

8. Drizzle the yogurt sauce over the tacos.

9. Serve hot.

Cooking Time: 20 minutes

21. Chickpea and Avocado Sandwich:

This vegetarian sandwich is a healthy and satisfying option for the beach.

Ingredients:

- 1 can of chickpeas, drained and rinsed

- 1 avocado, mashed

- 1/4 cup of chopped red onion

- 1/4 cup of chopped fresh cilantro

- 2 tablespoons of lime juice

- Salt and pepper

- 4 whole wheat bread slices

- 4 lettuce leaves

Instructions:

1. Use a fork or potato masher to mash the chickpeas in a medium bowl.

2. Add the mashed avocado, red onion, cilantro, lime juice, salt, and pepper to the bowl.

3. Stir items thoroughly until mixed.

4. Toast the bread slices.

5. Place a lettuce leaf on each slice of toast.

6. Divide the chickpea and avocado mixture between the four slices of toast.

7. Add a second slice of toast to the top of each sandwich.

8. Serve immediately.

Cooking Time: 10 minutes

22. Mediterranean Pasta Salad:

This pasta salad is packed with fresh veggies and tangy feta cheese.

Ingredients:

- 8 ounces of whole wheat pasta

- 1 cup of cherry tomatoes, halved

- 1 cucumber, chopped

- 1/2 red onion, thinly sliced

- 1/2 cup of pitted kalamata olives

- 1/2 cup of crumbled feta cheese

- 2 tablespoons of olive oil

- 2 tablespoons of red wine vinegar

- 1 tablespoon of Dijon mustard

- 1 clove of garlic, minced

- Salt and pepper

Instructions:

1. As directed on the packaging, cook the pasta.

2. Rinse the cooked pasta under cold water and drain well.

3. In a large bowl, combine the cooked pasta, cherry tomatoes, cucumber, red onion, kalamata olives, and feta cheese.

4. Olive oil, red wine vinegar, Dijon mustard, garlic, salt, and pepper should all be combined in a small bowl.

5. Toss the salad with the dressing after pouring it over it.

6. Serve chilled.

Cooking Time: 30 minutes

23. Turkey and Hummus Wrap:

This wrap is a great option for a quick and easy beach lunch.

Ingredients:

- 1 whole wheat tortilla

- 3 slices of deli turkey

- 2 tablespoons of hummus

- 1/4 cup of shredded carrots

- 1/4 cup of shredded lettuce

- 1/4 cup of diced cucumber

Instructions:

1. On a spotless surface, lay the tortilla out flat.

2. Spread the hummus evenly over the tortilla.

3. Add the slices of turkey to the centre of the tortilla.

4. Top the turkey with shredded carrots, lettuce, and cucumber.

5. Roll up the tortilla tightly.

6. Serve immediately.

Cooking Time: 5 minutes

24. Greek Yogurt and Berry Parfait:

This refreshing parfait is perfect for a beach breakfast or snack.

Ingredients:

- 1 cup of plain Greek yogurt

- 1 tablespoon of honey

- 1/2 teaspoon of vanilla extract

- 1/2 cup of mixed berries (such as strawberries, blueberries, and raspberries)

- 1/4 cup of granola

Instructions:

1. In a small bowl, whisk together the Greek yogurt, honey, and vanilla extract.

2. In a serving glass or jar, layer the Greek yogurt mixture, mixed berries, and granola.

3. Up until the glass or jar is filled, keep layering.

4. Serve chilled.

Cooking Time: 5 minutes

25. Grilled Shrimp Skewers:

These grilled shrimp skewers are a delicious and easy beach dinner.

Ingredients:

- 1 pound of peeled and deveined big shrimp

- 2 tablespoons of olive oil

- 2 cloves of garlic, minced

- 1 teaspoon of paprika

- 1/4 teaspoon of cayenne pepper

- Salt and pepper

- 4 wooden skewers

Instructions:

1. To keep the wooden skewers from burning on the grill, soak them in water for at least 30 minutes.

2. Grill or grill pan should be heated to medium-high.

3. In a medium bowl, whisk together the olive oil, garlic, paprika, cayenne pepper, salt, and pepper.

4. Toss the shrimp in the marinade after adding them to the bowl.

5. Thread the shrimp onto the soaked skewers.

6. The shrimp should be pink and cooked through after grilling them for two to three minutes on each side.

7. Serve immediately.

Cooking Time: 15 minutes

26. Quinoa and Black Bean Salad:

This protein-packed salad is perfect for a beach lunch or dinner.

Ingredients:

- 1 cup of quinoa

- 1 can of rinsed and drained black beans

- 1 red bell pepper, chopped

- 1/2 red onion, chopped

- 1/2 cup of chopped fresh cilantro

- 2 tablespoons of olive oil

- 2 tablespoons of lime juice

- 1 teaspoon of cumin

- Salt and pepper

Instructions:

1. As directed on the package, prepare the quinoa.

2. The cooked quinoa, black beans, red bell pepper, red onion, and cilantro should all be combined in a big bowl.

3. Mix the olive oil, lime juice, cumin, salt, and pepper in a small bowl.

4. Toss the salad with the dressing after pouring it over it.

5. Serve chilled.

Cooking Time: 25 minutes

27. Veggie and Hummus Sandwich:

This sandwich is a tasty and healthy option for a beach lunch.

Ingredients:

- 2 slices of whole grain bread

- 2 tablespoons of hummus

- 1/4 avocado, sliced

- 1/4 cup of sliced cucumber

- 1/4 cup of sliced bell pepper

- 1/4 cup of baby spinach

Instructions:

1. Toast the bread slices.

2. Spread the hummus evenly over one slice of toast.

3. Top the hummus with avocado, cucumber, bell pepper, and baby spinach.

4. Add the second piece of toast to the top.

5. Serve immediately.

Cooking Time: 5 minutes

28. Watermelon Salad with Feta and Mint:

This refreshing salad is a perfect beach side dish.

Ingredients:

- 4 cups of cubed watermelon

- 1/2 cup of crumbled feta cheese

- 1/4 cup of chopped fresh mint

- 2 tablespoons of olive oil

- 1 tablespoon of lime juice

- Salt and pepper

Instructions:

1. The cubed watermelon, feta cheese, and fresh mint are all combined in a big bowl.

2. Mix the olive oil, lime juice, salt, and pepper in a small bowl.

3. Toss the salad with the dressing after pouring it over it.

4. Serve chilled.

Cooking Time: 10 minutes

29. Tuna and White Bean Salad:

This protein-packed salad is a great option for a beach lunch.

Ingredients:

- 1 can of tuna, drained and flaked

- 1 can of white beans, rinsed and drained

- 1/2 red onion, chopped

- 1/2 cup of chopped fresh parsley

- 2 tablespoons of olive oil

- 1 tablespoon of lemon juice

- Salt and pepper

Instructions:

1. In a large bowl, combine the tuna, white beans, red onion, and fresh parsley.

2. Mix the olive oil, lemon juice, salt, and pepper in a small bowl.

3. Toss the salad with the dressing after pouring it over it.

4. Serve chilled.

Cooking Time: 10 minutes

30. Grilled Vegetable Skewers:

These colourful skewers are a great way to get your veggies in while enjoying the beach.

Ingredients:

- 1 red bell pepper, chopped

- 1 yellow bell pepper, chopped

- 1 zucchini, chopped

- 1 red onion, chopped

- 1/4 cup of olive oil

- 1 tablespoon of balsamic vinegar

- 2 cloves of garlic, minced

- Salt and pepper

Instructions:

1. To keep wooden skewers from burning on the barbecue, soak them in water for 30 minutes.

2. Grill or grill pan should be heated to medium-high.

3. Mix the olive oil, balsamic vinegar, garlic, salt, and pepper in a medium bowl.

4. Toss the chopped vegetables with the marinade in the basin after adding them.

5. Thread the vegetables onto the soaked skewers.

6. Grill the skewers for 2-3 minutes per side, or until the vegetables are charred and tender.

7. Serve immediately.

Cooking Time: 20 minutes

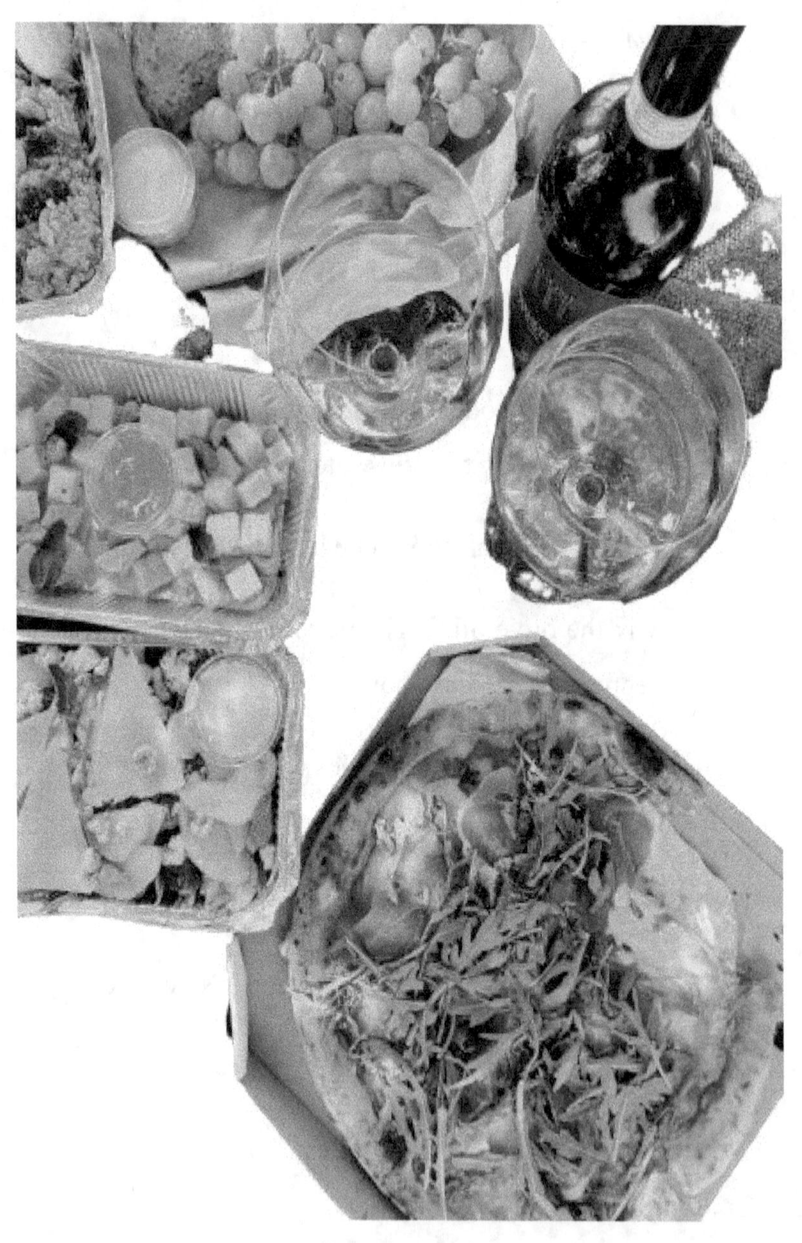

CONCLUSION

In conclusion, the Beach Body Diet is a popular diet plan that has gained a lot of attention in recent years. The diet plan is centred around the idea of eating whole foods, eliminating processed foods, and consuming a balanced amount of macronutrients.

One of the key features of the Beach Body Diet is that it encourages people to eat a wide variety of foods. This is important because it helps to ensure that people are getting all of the nutrients they need to maintain optimal health. In addition, the diet plan emphasizes the importance of consuming a balanced amount of macronutrients, which includes carbohydrates, protein, and healthy fats.

Another important feature of the Beach Body Diet is that it encourages people to avoid processed foods. This is important because processed foods are often high in unhealthy fats, sugar, and calories, which can contribute to weight gain and other health problems.

The Beach Body Diet also encourages people to exercise regularly.

Exercise is an important part of any weight loss or health plan because it helps to burn calories and build muscle. In addition, exercise can help to reduce stress, improve mood, and promote overall well-being.

Overall, the Beach Body Diet is a well-balanced and healthy diet plan that can help people achieve their weight loss and health goals. However, it is important to remember that everyone's nutritional needs are different, and what works for one person may not work for another. A healthcare practitioner should always be consulted before beginning a new diet or exercise regimen.

It is also important to remember that while the Beach Body Diet can be effective for weight loss and improving overall health, it is not a magic solution. In order to achieve lasting results, it is important to make lifestyle changes that are sustainable and realistic for the long term.

In conclusion, the Beach Body Diet is a healthy and balanced diet plan that can help people achieve their weight loss and health goals.

However, it is important to remember that there is no one-size-fits-all approach to nutrition and that it is always a good idea to consult with a healthcare professional before starting any new diet or exercise program. With dedication, hard work, and a commitment to a healthy lifestyle, anyone can achieve their desired level of health and fitness.